HOW TO KNOW IF A LOVED ONE IS USING DRUGS

LEARN WHAT TO DO TO HELP END DRUG ABUSE

JOHN GIANETTI

CONTENTS

INTRODUCTION

It is not a good feeling when you suspect a loved one is doing drugs. This book will provide you with very helpful tips and strategies to find out if someone is using drugs, and what to do if they are using drugs.

1
___

THE BASICS OF DRUG ADDICTION

Before you can manage to help your loved one overcome his or her drug addiction, it is important that you first equip yourself with the knowledge about how this condition works, and how it affects patients.

Drugs, in the general sense, are not necessarily addictive. A lot of people find them useful, whether it's for improving their performance in sports, treating certain medical conditions, or just for the sheer pleasure that they give when you take them. Drugs provide comfort and pleasure to those who take them, relieving a person of the symptoms of their illnesses and sometimes, giving them positive feelings which can encourage them to live their lives better and exhibit their full potential. However, there is a fine and blurry line between using drugs regularly and abusing their use. This fine line can vary depending on the case, and some people tend to succumb to drug abuse faster than others.

When we talk about drug abuse, we do not just consider how much drugs are consumed. This deals more of how it actually affects the life of a person. Is the use of the drug beneficial, or is it starting to do harm? Being addicted to the use of drugs is one thing, but if it starts to affect you and your relationship with others in a negative way, that is where the problem begins.

Drug abuse is a condition that heavily affects the brain of the patient. If a person becomes abusive, the drugs can actually do big changes with how a person thinks, feels and behaves by disrupting the brain's processes involving processing, sending and receiving information from the nerve cells. Drugs can do this in two ways: first, it can affect the region of the brain responsible for providing positive emotions or rewarding sensations, exaggerating their effects upon taking the drug; or second, by copying the structures of the brain's chemical messengers.

Marijuana and heroin have the ability to do this since their structures are almost similar to the neurotransmitters found in the brain, and because of this, they can "trick" the active receptors and nerve cells into sending the wrong messages to the brain. On another hand, there are also drugs that can mess or completely stop the recycling system of the brain chemicals, triggering the massive production of neurotransmitters. These drugs, such as cocaine and meth-amphetamine, disrupt the brain's normal functions and change most of the communication patterns in the nervous system.

Directly or indirectly, drugs can affect the brain in many ways, especially its reward system. An important chemical found in the brain responsible for feelings of pleasure, emotion, control movement and motivation: dopamine is significantly affected by the presence of drugs in the body through over stimulation, therefore making the brain *want* to repeat the use of the drug. If the patient does succumb to the use of these drugs, the brain reduces the production of dopamine receptors as a response, forcing the patient to consume more drugs in order to "stabilize" the dopamine levels and its functions. Long-term use can have serious effects not just on the dopamine levels, but also in other parts, circuits and chemicals in the brain. Drugs can even go as far as affecting regions of the brain responsible for judgment, decision-making, behavior, memory and learning.

A person's susceptibility to drugs can be affected by numerous factors. These factors can include the following:

- **Genes.** Drug addiction can also be hereditary. If a close family member such as a parent has a history of drug abuse, it is likely that the trait will be passed on to the children.

- **Environment.** A person who lives in a place where drug abuse is abundant is more likely to become affected by it.

- **The patient's mental health.** There are traumatic experiences that can trigger addiction in a person. These can include physical or sexual abuse, as well as neglect. People who show signs of depression have a bigger chance of becoming addicted to drugs. In addition to depression, anxiety and other mental disorders related to these can affect a person's tolerance towards drug abuse.

- **The manner of taking the drugs** is another
  factor that is considered when probability of
  addiction is discussed. The drug itself can
  contribute to its addiction factor. Drugs that are
  taken through smoking or through injection can
  become more addicting than other types of
  drugs, because these are taken directly by the
  body.

DRUG ABUSE IS a type of mental condition which can have serious effects on the person's mind and body. Although we can say that the person's initial consumption of the drug is voluntary, his control over his intake will eventually be reduced, and he will lose his ability to make the right decisions, choices, and self-control. The longer the person uses drugs, the effects become more severe until such a point comes that the drug itself is controlling the mind of the patient, making the impulses stronger.

This condition is not something that the patient can handle by himself. It is easy enough for the friends and family of the patient to say that it is just a matter of willpower and if he really wanted to quit, he can – however, this is not the true case.

DRUG ADDICTION IS MORE than just a matter of willpower. Science has allowed us to understand further on what happens inside the brain of a drug addict, and from the information gathered by research we can conclude that drug abuse is something that cannot be battled alone. The big neurological changes that happen to a drug addict are so drastic that finding the courage to stop their addiction can become extremely difficult, if not utterly impossible.

Luckily, treatment and medication is available to those people who want to combat their addiction. On a normal case, doctors would look for any underlying case which may have triggered the person's abuse, and then try to work those out until the person makes a full recovery. Medication is not the only thing a patient needs, however – family support is important as well.

SYMPTOMS TO LOOK OUT FOR

Do you have a suspicion that your loved one is abusing drugs? Does this worry you? Are there any changes that you noticed in him or her? As someone who cares, it is only normal for you to feel these things towards your loved one, regardless if he or she is your relative or friend. You can tell by how your loved one acts if he/she is a drug addict or not.

Symptoms of drug abuse must never be ignored. You should not just sit back and hope that these symptoms will just leave. If left untreated, the symptoms will get worse and will eventually lead to total drug dependence. Early on, it is important that you recognize these warning signs and symptoms.

If you worry that your loved one may be undergoing drug abuse, here are some signs of warning that you need to keep a look out for:

- Drug abuse symptoms affecting the overall physical health of the patient:

- There is obvious deterioration in how he appears.
- You may find that your loved one's belongings, including himself (body and breath) have an unusual smell
- Pupils appear to be smaller or larger than they are supposed to be, and the eyes are bloodshot.
- Your loved one has had significant weight loss
- There is change in sleep patterns and in appetite
- You have noticed that he tends to have frequent nosebleeds. These can be related to drugs that are snorted, for example cocaine or methamphetamine.
- He experiences seizures, even though he comes from a family that has no history of epilepsy
- Instances when he has accidents, injuries or bruises but he does not know how he got it in the first place.
- Unstable or impaired coordination. He may also experience tremors, shakes or may talk in a slurred or incoherent manner

- Changes in the behavior or people with drug abuse
- Sudden drop in work performance or in class attendance. They may exhibit a sudden loss in interest in participating in activities they enjoyed before, such as in their hobbies, exercise or sports. Motivation to do anything is obviously decreased
- If your loved one is a student, a decline in grades,

a sudden tendency to skip classes and often getting in trouble in school can be signs

- Tendency to steal or borrow money from you or from other family members. You may notice that money is missing from your wallet most of the time, as well as other valuables or prescription drugs stocked in your home
- You have received complaints from teachers, supervisors, co-workers or classmates concerning your loved one
- Your loved one gets into fights with either you or other members of the family more often, mostly because of clashes with family values or beliefs
- Tendency to act as if he is alone in the world. Most of the time you may notice that your loved one wishes to be alone. He or she may also have suspicious or secretive behaviors
- Your loved one is now more preoccupied with a lifestyle that is related to his or her drug abuse, which reflects in the way he dresses and in the music he listens to.
- He tends to avoid eye contact with anyone for as much as possible. He now also demands for more privacy and tends to lock his room and always keep to himself
- There is a sudden change in the people that make up his friendship circles. There are also changes in his hobbies and places where he hangs out
- Uses products with strong scents such as air fresheners, perfumes or incense to hide the smell of drugs or smoke

- In addition, your loved one also uses eye drops to hide his bloodshot eyes

- Psychological warning signs of drug addiction
- Sudden mood swings, shown in laughing at nothing, sudden irritability or angry outbursts
- Drastic and sudden change in attitude or personality
- Gives off a "spaced out" or lethargic appearance. Finds that he cannot focus on one thing for a long time and is not motivated to do anything
- There are periods when he is agitated or hyperactive
- For no reason he appears to be anxious, fearful, paranoid or withdrawn

SIGNS AND SYMPTOMS of Drug Addiction

Tolerance

This simply means that the need for more drugs gets stronger as time progresses. This can be checked by asking the patient if he needs to drink more to get the same effect that he used to have for lesser intake before.

WITHDRAWAL

When the effects of the drugs slowly wear off, the patient may experience symptoms of withdrawal. These include jumpiness or anxiety; nausea, sweating or vomiting; trembling or shakiness; fatigue, insomnia, headache and loss of appetite; irritability and depression. If the patients requires the intake of more drugs to overcome the symptoms of withdrawal, this may be a sign of addiction. In much more severe cases, the withdrawal symptoms can become life-threatening and may include seizures, hallucinations, confusion, agitation and fever. If these symptoms are felt by the patient, they should be immediately taken care of by a specially trained physician specializing in dealing with drug addicts.

Losing Control

Even if the patient tells himself multiple times that he will cut back on his drug consumption, or that he will not take drugs this time, he still does and would go beyond than what he intended initially

INABILITY TO STOP Drug Use

The patient has a persistent desire to stop or cut down his drug use, but all the efforts that he has made so far have proven to be unsuccessful

NEGLECT OF ACTIVITIES Other Than Those Involving Drugs

The patient may find that he now spends less time doing the things that used to occupy his free time, such as his hobbies, bonding with friends and family and doing exercises like jogging or going to the gym because of his drug use.

DRUG USE TENDS TO Take A Greater Time, Focus and Energy

The patient finds that he is more often preoccupied with thoughts concerning drugs, using it or recovering from the effects that they bring. There are only a few involvements in the community or society, or interests that do not involve drugs.

USE OF DRUGS *Still Go On Even With The Full Knowledge Of Its Side Effects*

The patient is fully aware of what the drug is doing to his body, but he/she still continues using it. For example, he realizes that the addiction is negatively affecting his job performance, doing damages to his relationship with his partner and causing serious physical and mental damages to his body.

3

COPING WITH YOUR LOVED ONE

A long with the physical and mental problems that drug addiction brings to a person, it can also do serious harm on the family of the addict. There no available statistics to show how much damage drug addicts have caused their families. However, there are things that you can do in order to cope with the stress when one of your loved one suffers from drug addiction and abuse. These range from educating yourself about the condition to establishing boundaries.

- The best place to start in coping with your loved one is by understanding the condition he is in. Keep in mind that drug addiction is a disease. There are factors that drug abuse has in common with illnesses such as cancer, diabetes and heart disease – all of them are chronic diseases that have roots coming from environmental and genetic causes. Addiction is not about strength of the patient's will. Just like how a person does not choose to have diabetes or cancer, your loved one did not choose to become a drug addict. Regardless of consequence, a person will continuously use drugs due to the changes that the drugs themselves make in the brain. When a person overuses drugs repeatedly, the pleasure system is overstimulated and in the process, they lose control of themselves and of their cravings.

- Understand that it was not your fault. Family members may blame themselves with what happened to their loved one, feeling that it is their fault and that they could have done something to stop the addiction from getting worse. This results in frustration, anger, helplessness and confusion. Knowing more about the condition can help you ease any anxiety that you may feel, as well as the stress that comes with dealing with your loved one. There are institutions that provide recovery meetings for families where a deeper understanding of drug addiction can be obtained by knowing that you are not alone in this situation.

- You should know these two terms: "detachment with love" and "enabling". These are concepts that families must learn concerning coping with a loved one's addiction. Enablers are family members who make up excuses for the behavior of their relative who causes chaos in the household, avoiding directly talking about the problem. In doing this, individual sense of self and personal boundaries is destroyed. Luckily there are ways for families to get over this, and one of those tools is "detaching with love". In this scenario, the addict is allowed to make mistakes and learn from those on his own at the allowance of the families themselves. This is in contrast of what many families do where the addict is shielded against the consequences brought about by their condition. The method bases itself on you loving the person yet detaching yourself from the disease in order to avoid the pain, stress and turmoil that come with it.

- Family therapy is important for this situation. Seek the help of a medical professional, specifically a therapist as a family in order to improve your connection with other members of the family. Therapy will provide the good platform where each family member can let out their inner frustrations and express their fears and any concerns they may have. Family therapy is also very important for the addict's children, in order to prevent them from going down the same path as their parent did.

- Stress and interpersonal problems are not the only ones that arise when a family member goes through drug addiction. The family finances can become affected as well, and not in a good way. That is why it is also important for you to seek the help of a financial counselor to help you make financial plans for you and your family's future. As you go over your family finances with your counselor, you may consider setting appropriate boundaries. This could mean the closing of shared accounts, refusing to lend money to the drug addict or you disassociating yourself from any financial burden or responsibility. You need to keep a close monitor of your finances. As a family member you are entitled to an annual financial report, because the earlier you see any surprise in your accounts, the better.

- Individual therapy sessions are not only important for the drug addict. If you are the spouse, partner or child of a drug addict, it is important that you go through therapy yourself in order to deal better with your situation and make sure that your mental health is also taken care of. Stress in dealing with a drug addict can be pretty heavy, and your mind will also need help. When you look for a therapist make sure that you go to someone who is accredited. You should also consider their methodologies and how much it would cost for you. However, the most important thing that you need to consider is how comfortable you are with him or her during your sessions.

- Open communication between you and your loved one is important. This helps in keeping and reestablishing family dynamics, during the addict's treatment and even after. This type of communication includes specific and clear statements. You should be the kind of person who is problem oriented and not person oriented. Always be honest with what you feel and be mindful and respectful of what others feel as well. In addition, with being a good communicator you should also be a good listener.

- To better help your family cope with the

addiction, do your best to keep everything as normal as possible. Your life does not necessarily need to drastically change when you find out that your loved one has drug addiction. Keeping normal family activities, or at least trying your best to keep them, will help you cope with the addiction. Although it is important that you recognize and accept the condition, it should not be the center of attention all the time.

- Be good to yourself. Sometimes when we take care and think of other people we often forget about ourselves and our own needs. Taking care of yourself both at a physical and an emotional level will not only help you, but will also help your family as well. Simple things like eating healthy, exercising and getting enough sleep every night will help your body cope better with stress. You could consider doing yoga which helps in reducing stress and in inducing relaxation in the mind and body, or if you want you can simply go out for a twenty minute walk out in a park.

4

THE DOS AND DON'TS OF COPING

There are things that as a relative or close friend of a person with drug addiction, you should do in order to make your coping better. Then, there are those things that you should avoid in doing at all times. Summarized here are the do's and don'ts when it comes to coping with a loved one that has drug addiction.

Do's

- Detach yourself from the condition. As what has been mentioned, practice detachment towards your loved one. Never become too obsessed with the condition of your family member. There are times that you just need to let things happen to your loved one in order for them to learn from experience. It is important for you to learn to let go so that your friend or relative with drug addiction will be able to see the consequences of his addictive actions.

- Recognize drug addiction as a disease. Remember that what your loved one is going through right now is the result of a medical condition affecting his mind, body, spirit and behavior. This is something that people can recover from. Keep in mind that it was not your loved one's intention to become an addict and that he is not doing this at you. The condition he is going through right now is beyond being a matter of willpower.

- Set some realistic demands and limits for you and for your loved one. Practice tough love towards him – this is the type of love which makes you make up your mind on what things you are going to accept concerning your loved one's addiction and what not to accept. However, as you set these expectations and limits remember to not feel like you are in control of your loved one's life. The act of changing must come directly from the addict and not from you. They require being sober for as much time as possible in order to maintain their recovery.

- Take it slow. It would be very impossible for you to tell what will happen in the future, so simply live a day at a time. When the going gets tough for you and for the rest of the family, remember the saying "this too shall pass". There are instances when you may feel like you are about to give up, but that is when your loved one will actually decide to make a change with his lifestyle and make a total turnaround.

- Take care of your family. In the period when the addiction is at its worse, and even if it is not, do not neglect the needs of other family members. If you have children, think about their needs as well and explain to them in terms that they can understand what is going on. Live your life as how you would live it without having to think of the addict regularly. Do not let his condition become the center of all your attention. Learn to enjoy life and have fun with your family and friends regardless if the addict participates or not.

- Look at yourself and check if there is anything about you that you can improve. Ask yourself what you need to learn, if there are any negative attributes that you may have concerning your character, and what are the good sides that you have as a person. Ask yourself what you need in order to be productive and happy in life.

Don'ts

- Do not make warnings or threats if you do not intend to carry them out anyway. Doing this will only weaken the limits you are enforcing and will only serve to reduce your credibility.

- Do not use harsh words, nor should you scold, ridicule or shame the addict in order to influence them out of the condition they are in. Keep in mind that the reason why they are addicted in the first place may come from depression due to lack of self-esteem or self-hatred, and arousing these kinds of emotions using your words will only increase the likelihood of taking drugs.

- Do not argue with the addict while he is under the influence. This will not give you anything but pure stress and frustration. In fact, you may even place yourself in a very dangerous situation if you do this. If there are things that you wish to talk about or point out to the addict, wait until he is sober before you talk to him, and use a level voice. Keep in mind that drug addicts will grab the opportunity of fighting in order to distract other members of the family from their condition.

- Do not fall for any reasons or alibis that the drug addict will tell you. The addict will only give you reasons why he has addiction so that it will appear to be reasonable to you, and thus valid. Remember that there is no good reason for someone to become an addict in the first place, and whatever your loved one tells you is nothing more than excuse rather than a really genuine explanation.

- Do not lie to the addict about what drug abuse can do to you, to other members of the family and to himself. Be completely honest, straightforward and calm when you tell them about it. Tell that family what is going on, but do not tell them in a way that will sound blaming, accusatory and heated.

- Do not hesitate to call the police when the need arises. At the same time, do not feel ashamed or guilty if you do this. Remember that it is not your intention to put anybody in harm and you are not a terrible person to do this. In addition, you may be doing this to stop the addict from doing something that can harm himself. What you need to remember is that the behavior of your loved one is not the result of what he feels towards you, but is a cry for help.

- Do not get the addict to stop his addiction for your sake. Reasons like "if you love me you will quit using drugs" normally do not work at all. Also, the addict needs to get himself sober and clean not for others but for himself because it is his life that is affected mainly.

- Do not cover up for your loved one with addiction. Let him experience whatever consequence his actions bring to him. Trying to make everything right for your loved one will only shield them from learning what they need to learn in order to wake up and try to solve the illness on their own.

- Do not encourage any activity that will motivate the addict into using drugs. In order to avoid having problems with drug addiction recurring for the addict, it is important for you and your family to avoid social functions like drinking parties or those that suggest drugging. The addict will become comfortable with these types of social gatherings over time, but in the period of recovery it is best that you stay away from them

- Do not be impatient. Recovery will take place in due time, and it will be a bit slow, so do not be impatient and look for immediate results. It will take time for you and your family to see significant changes in the addict's behavior. Enjoy the small improvements that happen and be happy with the small steps that the addict is making towards the direction of recovery.

5

___

HOW YOU CAN HELP

N ow that you have an idea with how you can cope
with your loved one's condition, it is now time for
you to know how you can help him or her in his
journey towards healing and recovery. There are many
things that you can do for your loved one, such as staging an
intervention or being there for them, and all of these are
listed below.

- Intervention. This is helpful in letting the
  members of the family to demonstrate to the
  addict how the condition is affecting their family.
  This should be done early on, so do not wait
  until everything has gone to a terrible situation
  before any action is made. The intervention can
  include the colleagues of the addict or members
  of a religious community (if the need arises).
  There can be a chance that the addict will be
  overwhelmed by the intervention, yet the point
  of this is not to put him in a defensive state so be

careful in which people you choose. Before this intervention even takes place, make sure to have a treatment plan already for the addict. This is important because the addict will not respond to the intervention if he does not know how he can get help or if he does not have a solid support from loved ones. Consider enrolling the addict in a treatment program even before the intervention begins, and even without the consent of the addict.

DURING THE INTERVENTION, those who will participate should provide a proof of how they have been negatively affected by their loved one's abuse of drugs. In most occasions, the people who stage the intervention choose letter-writing as a form of expressing their fears or concerns. Seeing how much the abuse damages the people around them is a strong motivator for the addict to change his ways. You should also plan on what consequences you are going to impose on your loved one if he decides not to cooperate with the intervention or with the recovery methods set up for him. However, make sure that you will follow through with whatever threats you make.

- Look for the right drug rehabilitation program. Before the intervention, it is important that you have already found one that will suit the condition of your loved one. In the case that intervention is not needed, you can help your loved one out in learning more about drug abuse and in looking for recommended plans for drug treatment. Support your loved one in his efforts

to recover and let him be in control of his own
rehabilitation

- Expect the Occurrence of Relapses. Since drug
  addiction is a chronic disease, it is something
  that can only be managed and not cured.
  Relapses are very likely to happen to your loved
  one, and this should not be viewed as a failure
  for the addict. In each instance that your loved
  one goes through an episode of relapse, he will
  need to go through treatment.

- Be There For Your Loved One. As someone who
  cares you should make the addict know that
  someone is there to help him out of his
  condition. Be there for them if they need you,
  even if the activity he wants is something that is
  not what you normally want to do. While you are
  with him, remember to always be positive.

AFTERWORD

Dealing and coping with a loved one who is doing drugs is challenging. I hope these strategies and tips covered in this book will serve you and your loved ones. I encourage you to keep this book handy and to use it as a guide if you ever suspect a loved one is using drugs.

www.ingramcontent.com/pod-product-compliance
Lightning Source LLC
Chambersburg PA
CBHW071533210326
41597CB00018B/2981